DAILA WEEKS

Stretch Smarter, Not Harder

50 simple at home stretches to enhance flexibility

This book was professionally typeset on Reedsy.
Find out more at reedsy.com

Contents

1

Introduction

Welcome to Stretch Smarter, Not Harder. I am so excited to write this book and have others experience the relaxation and benefits of stretching to increase your flexibility.

My name is Daila Weeks. A brief background of myself is that I have been a dancer since I was 3 years old, I am currently 26. Through my 23 years experience dancing I have learned and integrated many stretches into my daily routine. Stretching is a huge part of not only dance but any sport or athletics. Stretching is a form of movement I have found relaxes and grounds me. Performing stretches has increased my range of motion and over the years I have developed very high levels of flexibility. As an adult I have become an avid weightlifter. I find that in my personal experience I see more results from my workouts when I stretch consistently. Stretching has helped decrease my recovery time, soreness and tightness in my muscles. It continues to allow me to increase my flexibility as well as decrease physical pain. Most of the stretches I describe in this book I utilize in my daily stretch routine. It is important as with any other physical activity to stay consistent to see the best results. I recommend taking some stretches in this book from each body area and form a daily routine for yourself. I typically spend around

20 minutes a day stretching. If you are not able to fit a stretching routine into your everyday life I would suggest doing it at least 4-5 days a week. If you engage in other physical activities or workouts I think it is great to do a short warm up with a few stretches and after the workout do a longer more intense stretch session. Even if you are new to stretching or do not engage in other physical activities, these are 50 simple stretches that anyone can begin and see progress with if you continue and stay consistent. Be patient with yourself, everyone begins at their own level with flexibility and some of these stretches you will feel more intensely than others. My goal for this book is to make stretching more simple yet effective for anyone seeking to enhance their flexibility.

The benefits of increasing flexibility

Increasing flexibility has a wide variety of benefits that vary from person to person. Stretching can increase your blood flow and give you more energy. Your range of motion will also become enhanced which will decrease your chances of becoming injured through physical activity. Becoming more flexible can also improve how you perform in any sport or activity due to your muscles being able to move more fluidly and with less resistance. You may have different levels of flexibility on each side of your body so you want to aim to get to similar levels with each side. For example,If you do a stretch for your left hip,you want to do the same stretch for your right hip even if it is already more agile than the left. With this being said it is crucial to stretch your major muscle groups such as neck, back, shoulders, hips, and legs which all of those areas are included in this book. With these movements it is important to hold the pose to get the most out of the stretch. I will specify according to each exercise how long to stay in position. While stretching is not always comfortable it should not be painful but rather a feeling of tension and stretching of that muscular area. If you get into a stretch and you start experiencing pain, decrease the intensity or level to which you are performing the stretch until you get to a point in the movement where you feel slight tension and pulling but not the pain. If you are ever injured in any way that stretching could potentially affect such as a strained muscle, ankle sprain, etc. consult a doctor to ensure you are able to stretch that area before you continue stretching. Even if you do not have much time daily, creating a short 5-10 minute daily stretch routine can be very helpful in reaching your goal of increased flexibility. If you have more time in your schedule and want to aim for 15-25 minutes a day, then go for it. Follow the guide to stretch smarter, not harder and you will be on your way to a more flexible you! I am excited to begin this journey with you. Let's get started.

2

Neck Stretches

Tilted forward flexion- Begin standing or sitting and looking straight forward. You are now going to tilt your head to the right, still looking and facing forward then bring your chin to your chest. Once your chin is to your chest you are going to hold this for 10 seconds. Repeat this 5 times on the right side and move on to doing the same exercise but tilting your head left then chin to chest, also holding for 10 seconds and repeating 5 times.

Neck rotation- Begin standing or sitting looking straight forward. Now turn your head slowly to the right. Once your head is facing right, hold that position for 15 seconds then bring your head back to facing forward slowly. Now turn your head slowly to the left. Once your head is facing left, hold that position for 15 seconds and again bring your head back facing forward slowly. Do this exercise 5 times for each side.

Neck extension- Begin with a straight back either standing or seated. Looking forward, start to slowly bring your chin down to your chest. Once your chin is to your chest, hold that for 10 seconds. Slowly bring your head back up facing forward then slowly begin to extend your head straight back looking at the ceiling. Once you are looking at the ceiling hold that for 10 seconds. Slowly bring your head back facing center and repeat this exercise slowly moving the head down, straight and up 5 times.

3

Shoulder Stretches

Shoulder roll- Begin standing with your arms directly down by your sides, palms facing inward. Stand with your back straight and slightly tuck your chin. Slowly start to raise your shoulders up in a shrugging motion and bring them forward, down and around in a circular motion. While doing this your arms stay down by your sides, it is just your shoulders you are raising and circulating. Once you have made a full circle with your shoulders, repeat 3 times. Now you will repeat the same exercise but begin to circle your shoulders backwards, down and up to complete the circle this time. Do this 3 times slowly.

Shoulder cross arm swing stretch- Begin standing facing forward with your back straight and arms down by your sides. Bring your left arm up in front of you at a 90 degree angle to the floor. Now you are going to reach your left arm over to the right in front of you staying at 90 degrees. Once your left arm is in front of your right arm you are going to grab your left elbow with your right forearm and pull towards yourself until you feel the stretch in your left shoulder. Hold this pose for 30 seconds. Slowly bring your arms back down to the beginning position. Now time for the left side. Do the same exercise but you will extend your right arm and grab your right elbow with your left forearm and should feel the stretch in your right shoulder. Hold this side for 30 seconds before slowly coming back to center.

Reverse shoulder stretch- Begin standing with a straight back and feet shoulder width apart. Bring your hands behind your lower back/ glutes and clasp your fingers having your thumbs be facing down to the floor. Your pointer fingers should be closest to your back. Slowly begin to raise your arms with hands clasped behind your back as far up as you can feeling a stretching in the shoulders. Once you are as high as you can go, hold this for 30 seconds. Slowly bring your arms down and unclasp your fingers.

Thread the needle shoulder stretch- Begin by getting on the ground on all fours. You should be on your hands and knees facing downwards. Your hands should be in a straight line down from your shoulders and your knees should be in a straight line downward from your hips. Now you are going to bring your right arm under your left arm and begin to open your chest and torso to your left side. As you do this movement your left arm slides forward no longer being directly under your shoulder but out in front of it. When your right arm slides out to your left side your right palm is facing upwards. You should now be looking left with your right arm fully extended to the left of your body and your left arm stretching out in front of you. You should feel this stretch in your right shoulder. Once in position hold this pose for 30 seconds. Slowly release and get back into the beginning position. Now you are going to do this again but on the other side. Bring your left arm under your right arm and begin to open your chest and torso to the right. As you do this your right arm slides forward in front of your shoulder. Your left arm slides out to your right side and your left palm is facing upwards. You should now be looking right with your left arm fully extended to the right of your body and your right arm stretched out in front of you. You should feel this in your left shoulder. Hold for 30 seconds before slowly coming back to center.

4

Arm Stretches

Biceps stretch- Begin by standing sideways beside a wall with your right side of your body on the wall. Extend your right arm behind you somewhere between the height of your waist and shoulders. Now you are going to begin to turn your torso away from the wall feeling a stretch in your right bicep. Hold the pose for 30 seconds and return to the beginning position. Repeat this 1-2 times as needed. Now do the same stretch but with your left arm extending back and left side toward the wall and hold that side for 30 seconds repeating 1-2 times.

Triceps stretch- Begin facing forward standing with a straight back. Bring your right arm up and over your back with your right elbow facing upwards. With your left hand now push your right elbow back until you feel the stretch in your right tricep. Hold this for 10 seconds and repeat 3 times. Do the same for the left side with the left arm up and over your back and right arm pushing the left elbow back to feel the left tricep stretch. Hold for 10 seconds and repeat 3 times.

Wrist extension stretch (reverse clasp)- Begin standing with your left arm out 90 degrees in front of you with your palm facing out and fingers down. Take your right hand and pull your left fingers down and back to feel a forearm stretch. Hold this for 10 seconds and repeat 3 times. Do this with your right arm extended with your palm out and left hand pulling fingers down and back holding for 10 seconds and repeating 3 times.

5

Wrist Stretches

Wrist extension stretch- Begin standing with your left arm out at 90 degrees in front of you with fingers up and palm out. With your right hand pull your left fingers up and back feeling a left wrist stretch. Hold for 10 seconds and repeat 3 times. Do the same with the right arm extended with fingers up and palm out and left hand pulling right fingers back feeling a right wrist stretch. Hold for 10 seconds and repeat 3 times.

Prayer stretch- Begin facing forward and bring your hands up into a prayer position with palms touching facing each other in front of your chest. Raise both elbows to where they are almost straight across and push your fingers together to feel the stretch in both of your wrists. Hold this for 30 seconds and repeat as needed.

Wrist flexion stretch- Begin with your left arm out at 90 degrees in front of you with fingers facing down palm facing inward. With your right hand pull your left hand back and down towards you feeling a left wrist stretch. Hold for 10 seconds and repeat 3 times. Repeat on the right side holding your right hand out palm down and inward with left hand pulling right hand down and back. Hold for 10 seconds and repeat 3 times.

6

Hand Stretches

Clenched fist- Begin sitting down with hands on each leg with your palms upward. Clench your fingers together like a ball and slowly raise your wrists up off your legs bending your wrists back towards you. Hold this for 10 seconds then bring your wrist back down to legs spreading open your fingers. Repeat 3 times. Make sure to do this movement slowly and do not hold your fingers together too tight.

Thumb pull- Make a fist with your left hand with your thumb out and facing up. With your right hand pull your left thumb back until you feel a stretch. Hold for 10 seconds and repeat 3 times. Do the same for the right thumb with the left hand pulling the right thumb back and hold for 10 seconds. Repeat 3 times.

Alternate finger stretch- Bring your hands out in front of you with palms facing downward. Begin to spread your pointer and pinky finger apart simultaneously trying to keep your middle and ring finger together without separation. Repeat this slowly 5 times.

7

Back Stretches

Cat cow stretch- Begin by getting on all fours on the ground on your hands and knees. Place your hands directly under shoulders and knees under your hips. Take a deep breath inward as you bring your chest in. Raise your back upward scrunching your back in. Exhale that deep breath and extend your chest outward now arching your back out. Hold each of the 2 poses for 15 seconds and repeat the exercise 3 times.

Child's pose- Begin by getting on all fours on the ground on your hands and knees. Slightly begin to slide your hands forward and bring your back and glutes downward. Once in position while still having your palms down on the ground, try to slide down and back as far as you can to have your glutes resting by your feet. With your head and chest down, hold this pose for 30 seconds repeating 3 times.

Swinging fan stretch- Begin standing facing forward with arms down by your sides. Slowly start to rotate your torso left swinging your arms left then slowly rotate your torso right swinging your arms right. Do this back and forth for 30-45 seconds. You will feel this stretching and loosening up your back.

Seated spinal twist- Begin by sitting on the ground with a straight back and legs out straight in front of you. Bring your right leg up to where your right foot is aligned with your left knee or a little lower and cross your right foot over your left leg. Now take your left elbow and place it on the right side of your right knee. Your torso should now be facing right. Hold the elbow on the knee and and keep twisting the torso to the right feeling that back stretch and hold for 30-60 seconds. Come back to the beginning position and bring your left leg up to where your left foot is aligned or close to your right knee and cross your left foot over right leg. Now take your right elbow and place it on the left side of your left knee. Your torso should now be facing left. Hold that side for 30-60 seconds.

Open book stretch- Begin by laying on the ground on your back. Turn to your left side while keeping your legs,knees and feet together. Bend your legs slightly and extend your arms out in front of your face, palms facing each other and touching. Now lift your right arm up and over your body until it's in the same position as your left arm but on the right side of your body with your palm upward. While doing this keep your legs together and on the ground and left arm on the ground where it is. Once your right arm is extended over your body on the right side your back should now be almost completely on the ground feeling that back stretch. Hold this position for 30 seconds. Slowly bring the right arm back over to touch the left arm. Repeat this on the other side. Turn to your right side keeping legs together on the ground and extend your arms out. Now the left arm lifts up and extends over to the left side with your back almost completely on the ground again. Hold for 30 seconds and bring arms back together.

8

Chest Stretches

Above head chest stretch- Begin by standing with your back straight. Bring your hands behind your head with elbows facing directly outward. Pull your elbows back and bring the back of your shoulders together while keeping your fingers interlocked on the back of your head. Hold this stretch for 30-60 seconds.

Bent arm wall stretch- Begin standing beside a wall with your right arm touching the wall from the right elbow up to your right hand. Your elbow is aligned with your shoulder height with your arm facing upward, palm on the wall, fingers facing up. Stand with your feet apart with your right foot forward. Press your right arm into the wall while slightly twisting your torso to the left and turning your head left. Hold this for 20 seconds. Do on the opposite side now with your left arm up on the wall and left foot forward. Press your left arm into the wall and twist your torso and head to the right and hold for 20 seconds. Do this twice on each side.

Camel pose- Begin by getting on the ground on your knees with your back up straight facing forward with your hands down by your sides.

Now take your hands and reach behind you and grab the inside of your ankles (left hand left ankle,right hand right ankle). While grabbing your ankles arch your back and lean back to where your head is facing up at the ceiling. Push your chest out while you arch your back.Hold this pose for 20-30 seconds. Repeat as needed.

9

Core Stretches

Cobra pose- Begin by laying down on your stomach. You are going to keep your legs straight behind you with feet pointed. Raise your upper body up until your arms are extended out past your shoulders keeping your elbows close to your side and hands flat on the ground. Lift up and back as far as you can, arching your back and bringing your head up until you feel a pulling stretch in your core. Hold this pose for 20 seconds and repeat 3 times.

Obliques stretch- Begin standing facing front. Keep your feet shoulder width apart. Have your right arm bent with your hand resting on your hip. Bring your left arm over your head with your palm facing down. Reach over to the right side until you feel a stretching in your left oblique and hold this for 15 seconds. Repeat this on the other side having your left arm bent and left hand on hip and your right arm reaching over to your left side until you feel the stretching in your right oblique. Hold for 15 seconds and repeat twice on each side.

Seated side straddle stretch- Begin by sitting on the ground and spreading your legs apart as far as you can into a straddle. Now you are going to lift your left arm over your head and over to the right as if you are trying to grab your right foot. You can leave your right arm on the floor in front of you or place it on your left thigh.Reach as far right as you are able to and feel the stretch in your obliques. Hold this position for 30 seconds. Do the same on the other side reaching with your right arm over your head towards your left foot. You can rest your left arm on the ground or on your right thigh. Hold for 30 seconds and repeat on each side one more time.

10

Hip Stretches

Standing hip circles- Begin standing straight forward with feet shoulder width apart. Place your hands on your hips and bring your right knee up in front of you at about a 90 degree angle. Rotate your hip to the right in a circular motion moving your knee to the front,side, then back of you placing your foot on the ground after completing the circle. Do this movement slowly 3 times then do it again with circular motion in the opposite direction starting back,side, then front. After you've done this on the right 3 times, move to the left and do 3 forward circles with your left knee and hip slowly and then 3 backwards circles.

90/90 stretch- Begin sitting on the ground with your right leg in front of you and left leg behind you. Bend your right knee at 90 degrees to where your right foot is pointing left and your front leg is in bent v shape on the ground. Now bend your back left leg with your left foot facing right but the leg should not be bent as tight as your front leg . This bend should be a bigger v shape than the front leg. Keep both of your feet flexed and the soles of your feet facing side. Now hold this pose for 30 seconds trying to maintain your right glute on the floor and pressing your left glute as close to the floor as you can.

Repeat this stretch with your left leg forward and right leg back. Now your left glute should be on the floor and you are aiming to get that right glute as close to the ground as possible while holding for 30 seconds.

Lying figure-four stretch- Begin by laying down on your back. Bring your left knee up at a 90 degree angle then place your right foot over the left knee with the sole of the foot facing left and toes upward. Grab the back of your left thigh and pull towards you feeling a stretch and hold for 20 seconds. Now repeat this on the other side with your right knee at a 90 degree angle and place your left foot over your right knee with your foot facing right. Grab your right thigh and pull to hold for another 20 seconds. Do this twice on each side.

Pigeon pose- Begin seated with your right leg fully extended straight behind you and left leg forward bent as tightly and close to you as possible with the sole of your left foot facing right. Your left foot can be as close as possible to your right hip for this pose. Try to maintain a flexed left foot and right hip close to the ground. Hold this pose for 45-60 seconds feeling the left hip stretch. Repeat on the other side with right leg front and bent and left leg extended straight behind you. Bring your right foot to your left hip and hold for another 45-60 seconds.

Lunging hip flexor stretch- Begin by kneeling down with your right knee back with leg extended and have your front left leg bent in front of you with your left foot flat on the ground. Place your hands on your knees and bend forward until you feel a pulling stretch in your right hip. Hold the pose for 30 seconds. Now repeat on the other side with your right leg bent and foot flat on ground front and left leg kneeling extended back. Keep your hands on your knee bending forward again for 30 seconds.

11

Leg Stretches

Standing forward bend- Begin standing straight with feet together facing forward. Bend over forward and grab the back of your legs. Try to pull yourself into your legs as much as you can while keeping your legs straight and both feet on the floor. You will feel this stretch in your calf and hamstrings. Hold this pose for 30 seconds.

Quad stretch- Begin standing feet shoulder width apart with left hand on a wall for balance support. Now pick up your right foot with your right hand and pull your foot up to the back of your glutes/hamstring. You should feel a stretch in your right quad and hold this for 30 seconds. Now repeat on the other side with your left leg and with your right hand on the wall for balance and hold for 30 seconds.

Hamstring calf stretch- Begin by sitting on the ground with legs out directly in front of you. With feet flexed reach forward as far as you can aiming to grab your toes and pull them back towards you. If you can not reach your toes grab your feet and pull your chest forward as much as you can. If you can not reach your feet then grab as far down on your legs as you can and pull downward. Hold this position for 30 seconds.

Runner's lunge- Begin on the ground in a plank position facing down. Now slide your right leg in between your arms until it is directly under your shoulder at a 90 degree angle with your right foot flat on the ground. Extend your left leg back straight, balancing on the ball of your left foot. Place your hands on both sides of your front leg and press down to the ground until you feel the stretch. Hold this for 30 seconds. Repeat on the other side now with left leg forward and right leg back holding for another 30 seconds.

Supine hamstring stretch- Begin laying on your back with both legs straight in front of you on the floor. Lift your right leg up to where you can grab your toes and start pulling your leg towards you as far as you can while keeping your leg straight. If you are having trouble reaching your toes you can use a resistance band or towel. Hold the stretch for 30-45 seconds. Now repeat on the other side bringing the left leg up to grab your toes and pull as far as you can towards your face keeping the leg straight. Hold for 30-45 seconds.

Half splits- Begin on all fours. Bring your right leg forward between your arms and extend it straight as much as you can holding your weight in your front heel. Extend the left leg back bent at the knee with knee touching the ground and holding weight in the ball of the foot. Balance and hold your weight with your hands on each side of you. Exhale keeping your body facing forward and bend over as much as you can towards your front leg. Hold this for 30 seconds. Repeat now on the other side with the left leg forward and right leg back. Hold for another 30 seconds.

Front splits- Begin by getting into a low lunge position with your right leg forward and left leg back. With hands on either side of you for balance and support begin to slide out as far as you are able to with your front and back leg straight. Point your feet and get to the point where you feel the stretch and hold that position for 60 seconds. If you are able to fully sit in the front split, still hold it for the 60 seconds and focus on having hips on the ground centered and back up straight. Repeat on the other side with left leg forward and right leg back and hold for another 60 seconds.

Deep squat- Begin standing with feet spread apart past your shoulders. Bend down now into a squat position. Bring your elbows to the inside of your knees and hands together in a prayer position. Now push hands together and elbows out into your thighs so your legs are getting pushed outwards feeling a stretch in the hips. Hold this for 30 seconds.

Butterfly pose- Begin by sitting down with legs in front of you and bring the soles of your feet to meet together in the center. Now hold your feet and start to press your legs into the floor with your elbows. Once you have done this, begin to reach forward while keeping a long straight back. Now you should feel the stretch. Hold this pose for 30 seconds.

Supine straddle- Begin by laying down on your back and lift your legs up in front of you on a wall. Your glutes should be touching the wall with your back completely on the floor. Now spread your legs out as far as you can to each side and pull down on your thighs to ensure you are in as deep of a straddle as you can be. Once you're at the point where you feel a strong stretch hold this position for 60 seconds.

Frog pose- Begin by getting on the ground on your hands and knees. Now extend your knees outward as far as you are able to while bringing your feet straight behind your knees. Now try to bend forward as much as you can, having your hips be as close to the ground as possible with feet flexed. You will feel a strong stretch in the hips. Hold this pose for 30-45 seconds.

Straddle with reach- Begin sitting on the ground in a straddle position with your legs as far open and apart as you can go. Take your arms forward and center and pull yourself down as much as you can as if you are trying to bring your hands all the way forward and core on the floor. Once you have pulled as far forward as you can hold this for 60 seconds.

Middle split- Begin by standing and spread your legs out to the side, sliding them as far as you can placing your hands on the ground in front of you shoulder width apart for balance and support. Push your legs out to each side as far as you can, keeping them straight and in alignment with your hips. Once you are down as far as you can go hold this position for 60 seconds. If you are completely down into the split point your toes and focus on being in a straight alignment from hip to toe.

12

Foot Stretches

Toe raise, point and curl- Begin sitting in a chair with feet flat on the ground. Now extend your toes up where only heels are touching the ground hold for 5 seconds. Slowly bring them back down. Now point your toes as hard as you can slowly and hold for 5 seconds. Now curl your toes under your feet holding for 5 seconds and then roll them back flat on the ground. Repeat this 3 times.

Toe extension- Begin sitting in a chair with feet flat on the ground. Pick your right foot up and put it on your left thigh. With your right hand grab your toes and pull them back until you feel a stretch. Hold this for 10 seconds. Now do the same with your left foot on your right thigh and pull your left toes back until you feel the stretch and hold for 10 seconds. Do this 3 times on each side.

Toe splay- Begin sitting in a chair with feet flat on the ground. Now spread all of your toes out as far as you can. Hold the spread for 5 seconds and repeat 3 times.

13

Ankle Stretches

Ankle circles- Begin sitting with your legs out in front of you. Slowly rotate your ankles in a clockwise motion and slowly make a circle. Do this 5 times. Now slowly rotate your ankles in a counterclockwise motion slowly making a circle. Do this 5 times as well. Make sure it is just your ankle and foot moving that your leg remains still on the floor.

Standing heel lifts- Begin standing straight with legs shoulder width apart. Place your hands on your hips and lift your heels off of the ground. Once standing on the balls of your feet slowly lower the heels until the feet are back to flat. Do this in 2 sets of 15 raises.

14

Conclusion

I hope you have enjoyed reading this book as much as I enjoyed writing and creating it. Hopefully now you can confidently say you have learned how to stretch smarter, not harder. I wish you the best in your personal stretching and flexibility journey. Try to stay consistent and build your daily stretching routine that works for you from the stretches I have provided. I would greatly appreciate it if you would leave a review for this book. Thanks so much,

Daila

15

Resources

Mayo Clinic staff. (2023, November 18). *Stretching: Focus on flexibility*. Mayo Clinic. Retrieved November 28, 2023, from https://www.mayoclinic.org/healthy-lifestyle/fitness/in-depth/stretching/art-20047931

Neck exercises. (n.d.-b). The Bone and Joint Clinic Texas Healthcare Fort Worth. Retrieved November 28, 2023, from https://thcboneandjoint.com/educational-resources/neck-exercises.html

Minnis, G., DPT, & Bass, L. (2021, February 25). *Brush Your Shoulders Off with These 11 Shoulder Mobility Exercises*. GREATiST. Retrieved November 28, 2023, from https://greatist.com/fitness/shoulder-mobility-exercises#shoulder-mobility-vs-flexibility

Wilson, C. & SPE Medical Review Board. (2022, September 6). *Arm Stretches*. Shoulder Pain Explained. Retrieved November 28, 2023, from https://www.shoulder-pain-explained.com/arm-stretches.html

Forearm Stretches that Improve Your Flexibility. (n.d.). PT Linked. Retrieved November 28, 2023, from https://www.ptlinked.com/exerc

ise-program/forearm-stretches-that-improve-your-flexibility

The Healthline Editorial Team, & Minnis, G., DPT. (2019, May 14). *Stretches for Wrists and Hands* (F. Crooks, Ed.). Healthline. Retrieved November 28, 2023, from https://www.healthline.com/health/chroni c-pain/wrist-and-hand-stretches#building-strength

Stinson, A., & Minnis, G., DPT. (2019, February 19). *How to stretch your hands and wrists.* MedicalNewsToday. Retrieved November 28, 2023, from https://www.medicalnewstoday.com/articles/324489#Wrist-a nd-hand-stretches

Dewar, M. (n.d.). *10 Back Flexibility Stretches To Improve Mobility & Performance.* FITBOD Blog. Retrieved November 28, 2023, from https://fitbod.me/blog/back-flexibility-stretches/

Williams, A. (2021, June 29). *Best Chest Stretches For Tight Chest Muscles.* O R I G Y M. Retrieved November 28, 2023, from https://origympe rsonaltrainercourses.co.uk/blog/best-chest-stretches-for-tight-chest-muscles

Lindberg, S., & Minnis, G., DPT. (2019, August 29). *How to Stretch Your Abs and Why It Matters.* Healthline. Retrieved November 28, 2023, from https://www.healthline.com/health/exercise-fitness/how-to-stretch-abs#examples-of-stretches

Core Static Stretching Routine. (n.d.). SPOTEBI Fitness & Nutrition. Retrieved November 28, 2023, from https://www.spotebi.com/worko ut-routines/core-static-stretching-exercises/

5 Core Stretches That Will Make Your Abs Feel Amazing. (n.d.). livestrong.com. Retrieved November 28, 2023, from https://www.live strong.com/article/355186-core-muscle-stretches/

Marturana Winderl, A., C. P. T., Millard, E., C. P. T. ,. R. Y. T., & Sgobba, C., C. P. T. (2023, November 7). *16 Hip Stretches Your Body Really Needs.* SELF. Retrieved November 28, 2023, from https://www.self.com/gall ery/hip-stretches-your-body-really-needs-slideshow

How to Do the Splits: Best Stretches and Safety Tips. (2022, May 6). DAILY BURN. Retrieved November 28, 2023, from https://dailyburn.com/ life/fitness/how-to-do-the-splits/

Goldman, R., & Minnis, G., D. P. T. (2020, May 5). *4 Leg Stretches for Flexibility.* Healthline. Retrieved November 28, 2023, from https://w ww.healthline.com/health/exercise-fitness/leg-stretches-flexibility# 3-HIIT-Moves-to-Strengthen-Hamstrings

Axtell, B., & Minnis, G., D. P. T. (2018, February 27). *9 Foot Exercises to Try at Home.* Healthline. Retrieved November 28, 2023, from https://w ww.healthline.com/health/fitness-exercise/foot-exercises

Hecht, M., & Morrison, W., M. D. (2019, May 28). *12 Stretch and Strength Moves for Ankle Mobility.* Healthline. Retrieved November 28, 2023, from https://www.healthline.com/health/ankle-mobility#ankle-circl es